The ABC's of CANCER

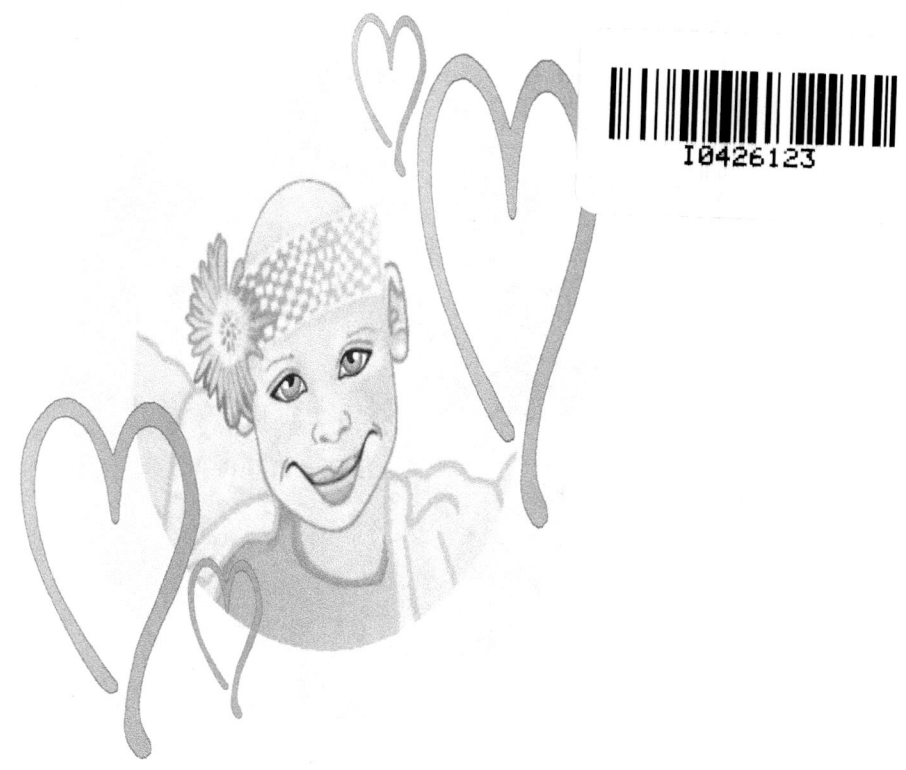

"According to Lilly Isabella Lane"

Author Terri Forehand

Illustrator Dawn M. Phillips

My name is Lilly Isabella Lane...Lil for short. I am nine years old. A few months ago, I was just a normal kid.

Then I got a fever. I had no energy to play or ride my bike or go to school. I just wanted to sleep.

My mom took me to the doctor, and now I know that I have a childhood form of cancer called Acute Lymphocytic Leukemia. Some kids might say it stinks, but that isn't how I look at things. This is what I have to say about it in my own words, especially to other kids who have cancer, too.

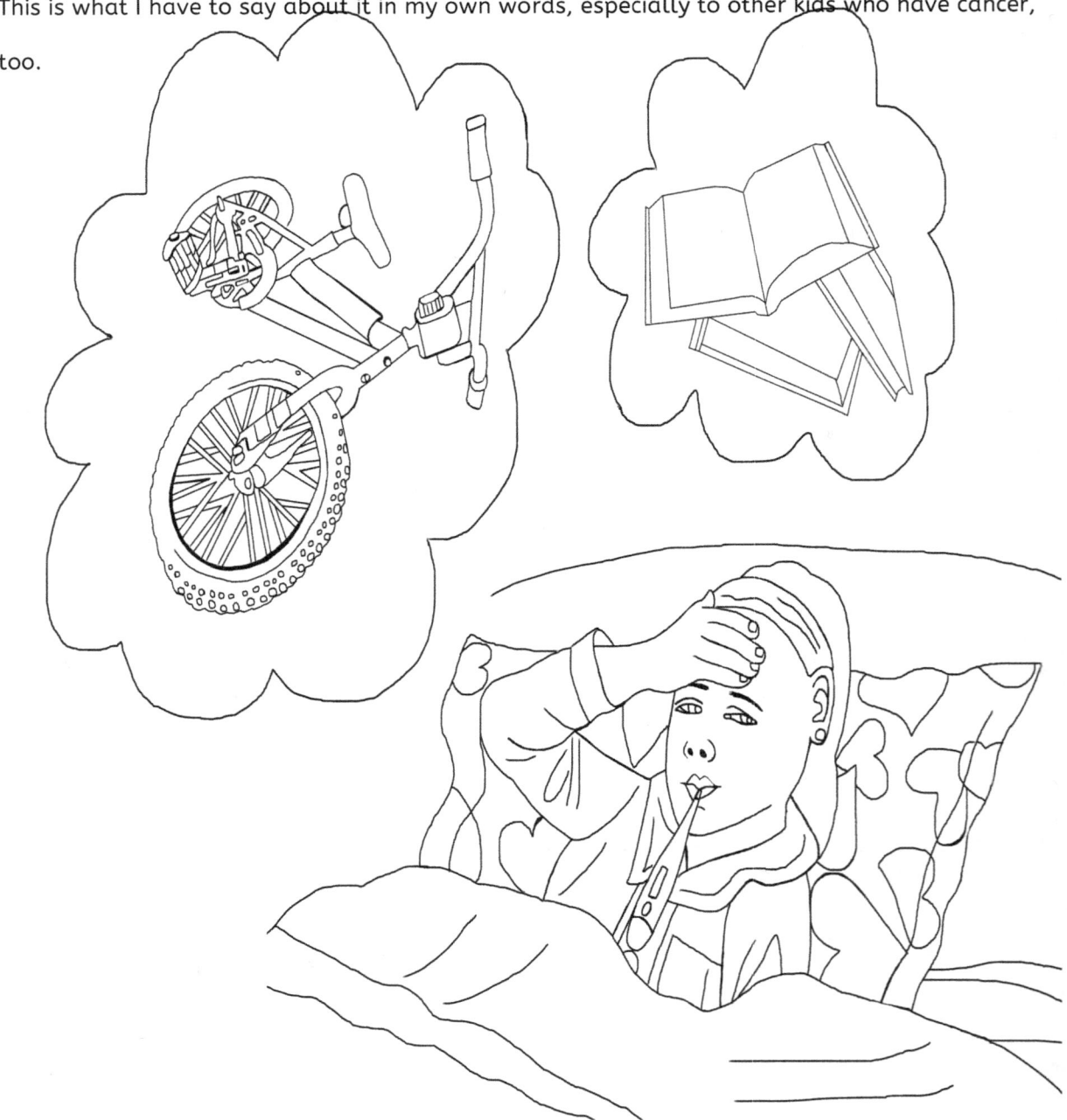

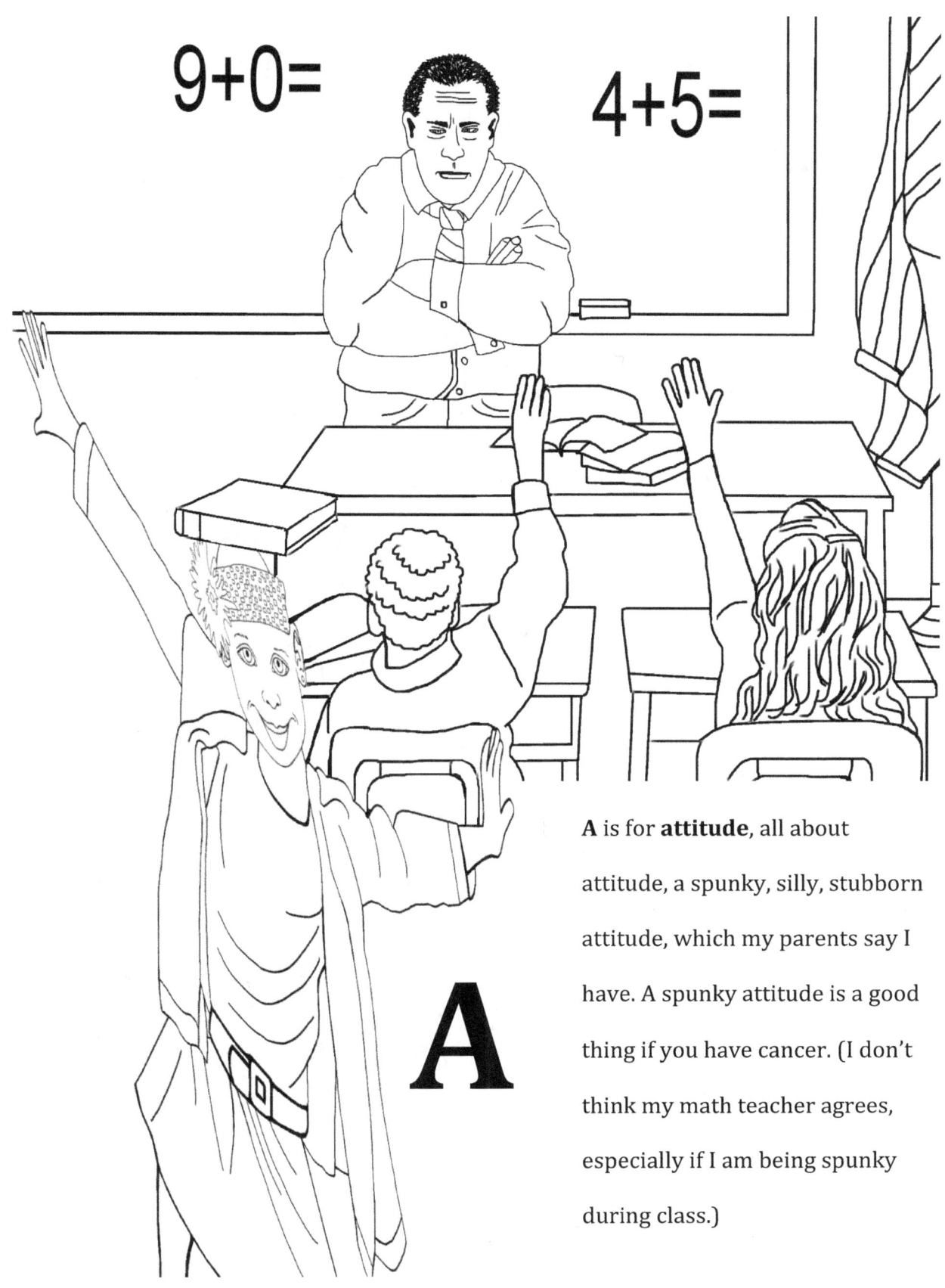

A is for **attitude**, all about attitude, a spunky, silly, stubborn attitude, which my parents say I have. A spunky attitude is a good thing if you have cancer. (I don't think my math teacher agrees, especially if I am being spunky during class.)

B is for **bald**. Bald is beautiful, and you don't get tangles. The treatment for my leukemia makes my hair fall out in clumps and patches. I asked my dad to shave my head bald...now no tangles. (He shaved his head, too, so he could look like me.)

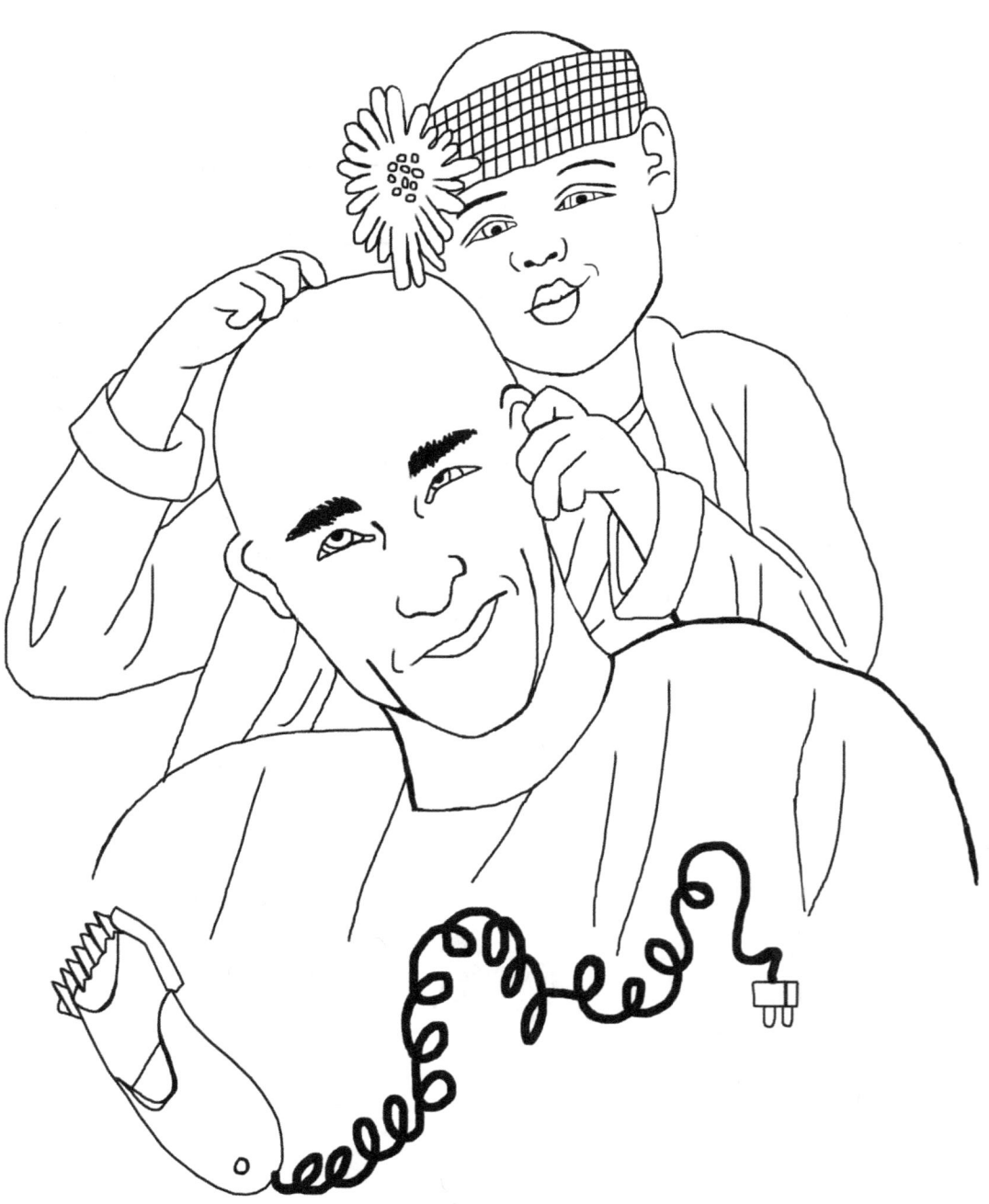

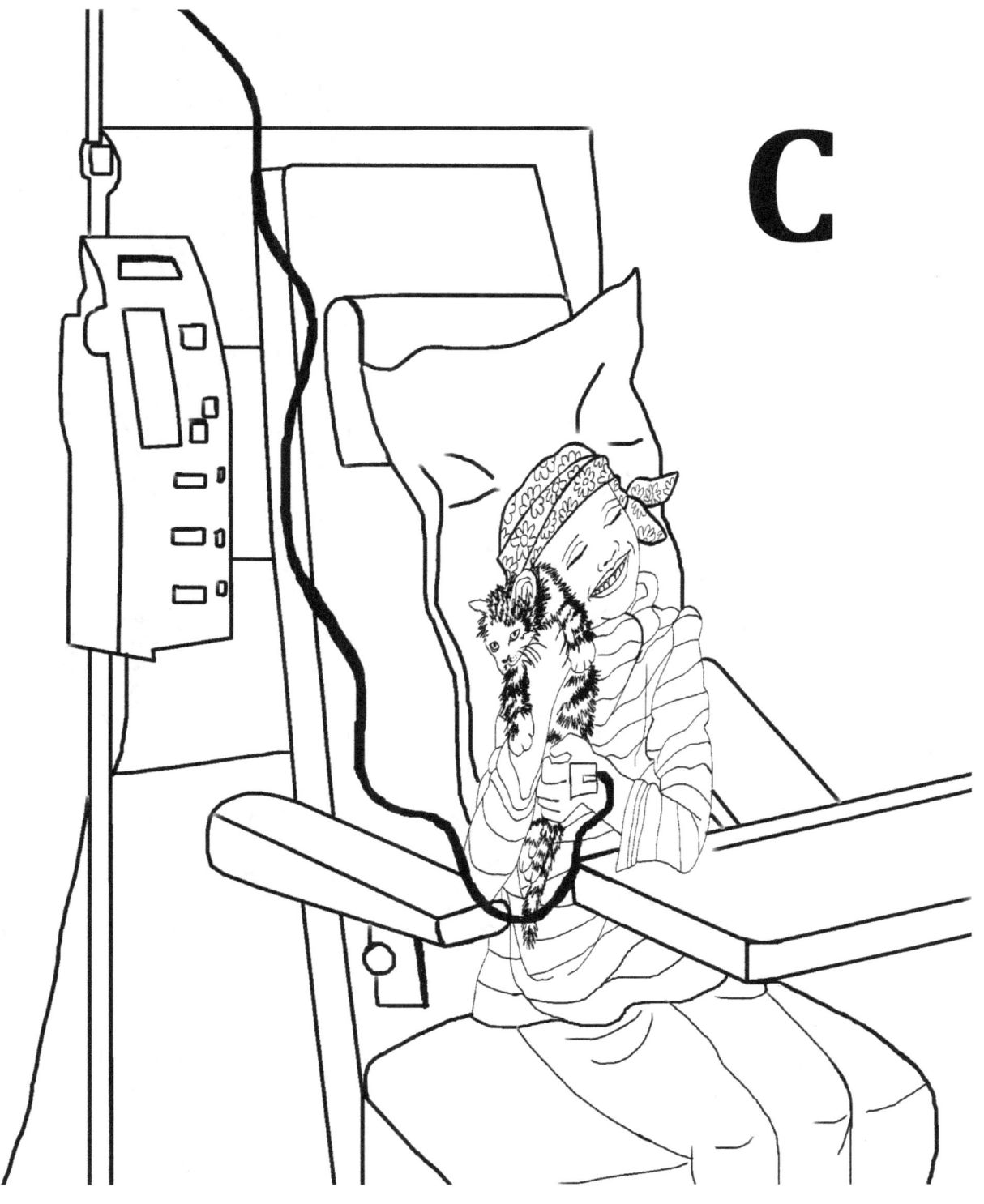

C is for **cancer**, **chemotherapy**, and **cuddling**. With cancer you have to take chemo, and

the chemo makes you feel crummy, but cuddling my cat helps.

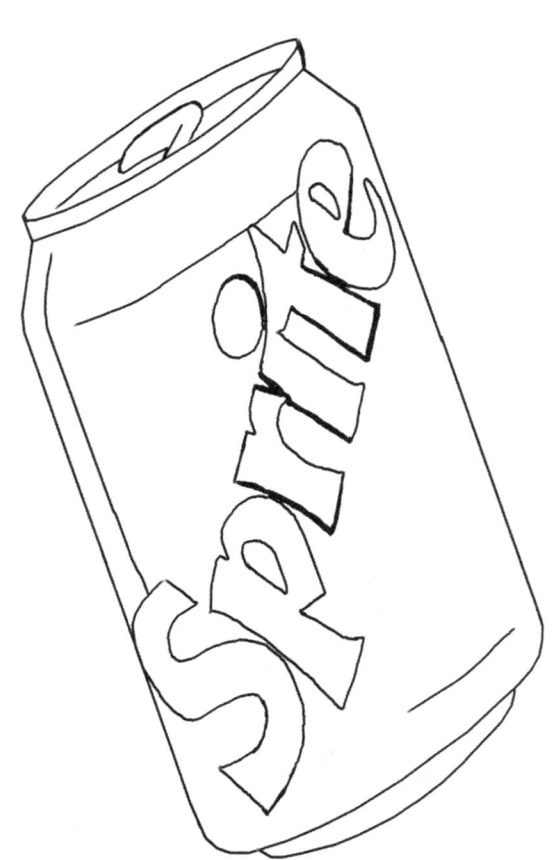

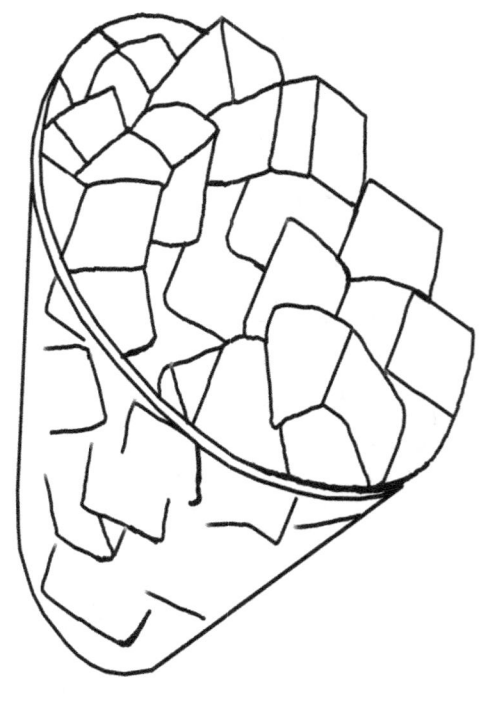

D

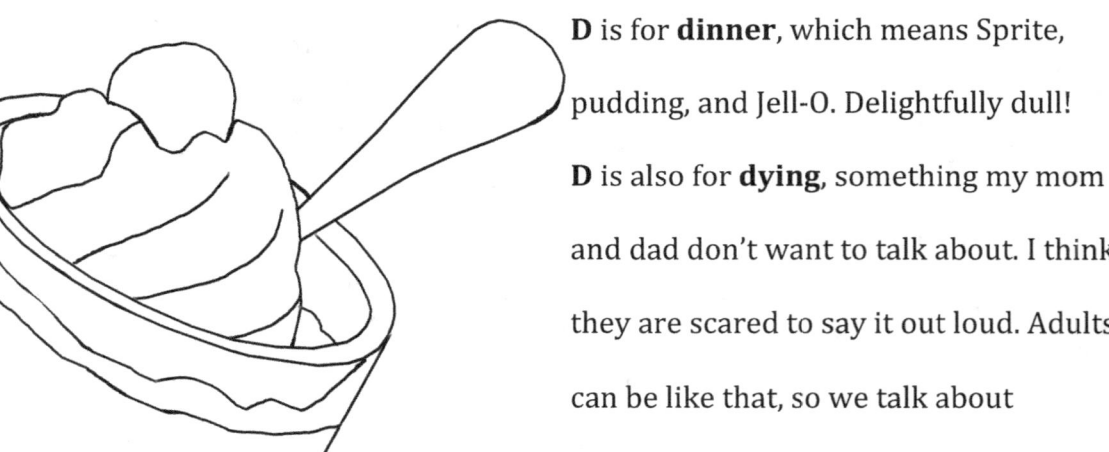

D is for **dinner**, which means Sprite, pudding, and Jell-O. Delightfully dull! **D** is also for **dying**, something my mom and dad don't want to talk about. I think they are scared to say it out loud. Adults can be like that, so we talk about something silly like ducks with feathers

E is for the **effort** of all of the doctors and nurses making me better. Thanks and thanks again. Love, Lilly.

E is also for **earrings**, bright shiny hoops, hearts, and stars, oh my. Earrings make my brown eyes sparkle.

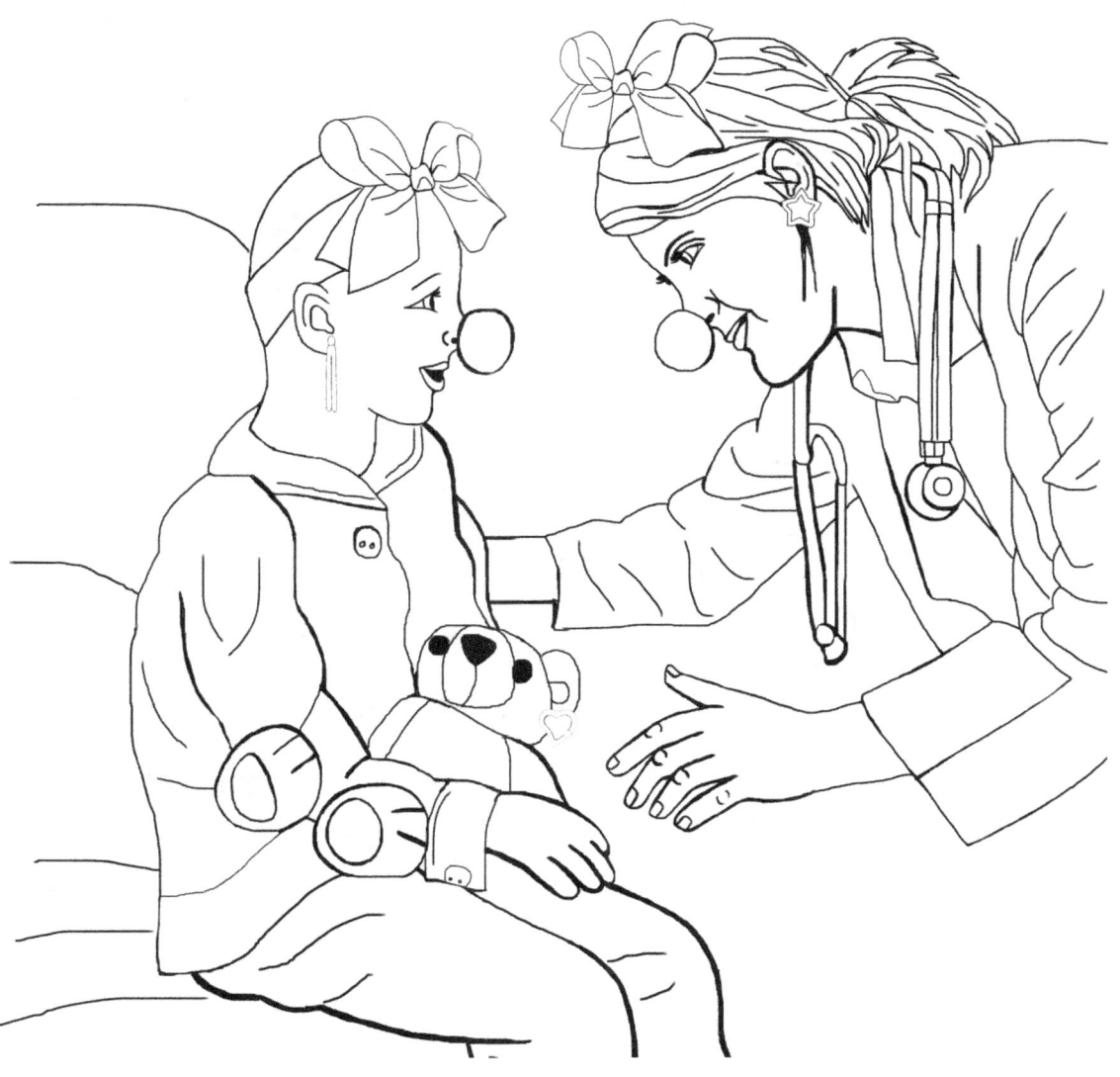

F is for **fun with friends**...silly, goofy, crazy fun, and forgetting you are kind of sick. Funny faces and dressing up kind of fun, face painting fun, and baking fudge cupcakes kind of fun.

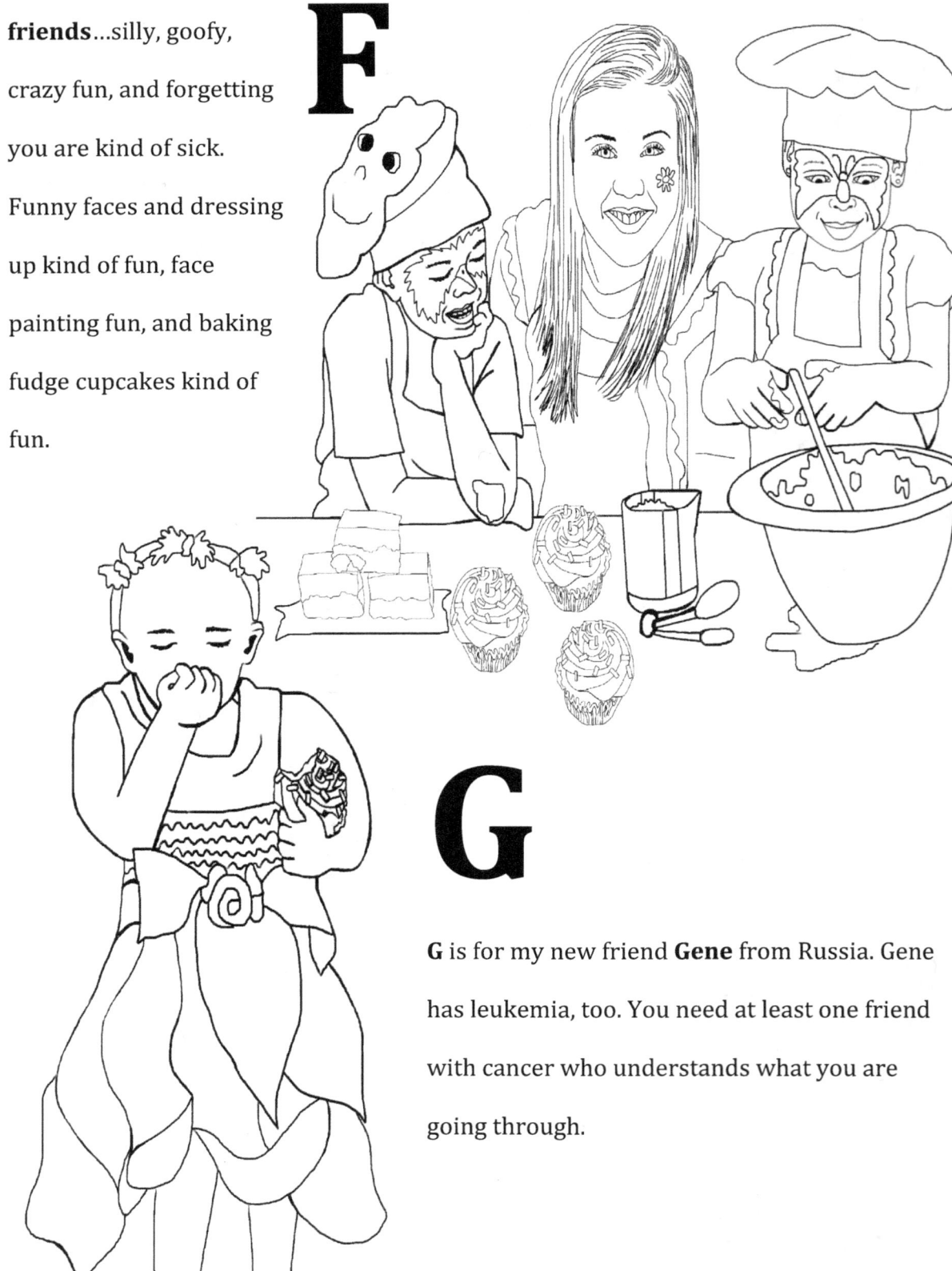

G is for my new friend **Gene** from Russia. Gene has leukemia, too. You need at least one friend with cancer who understands what you are going through.

H

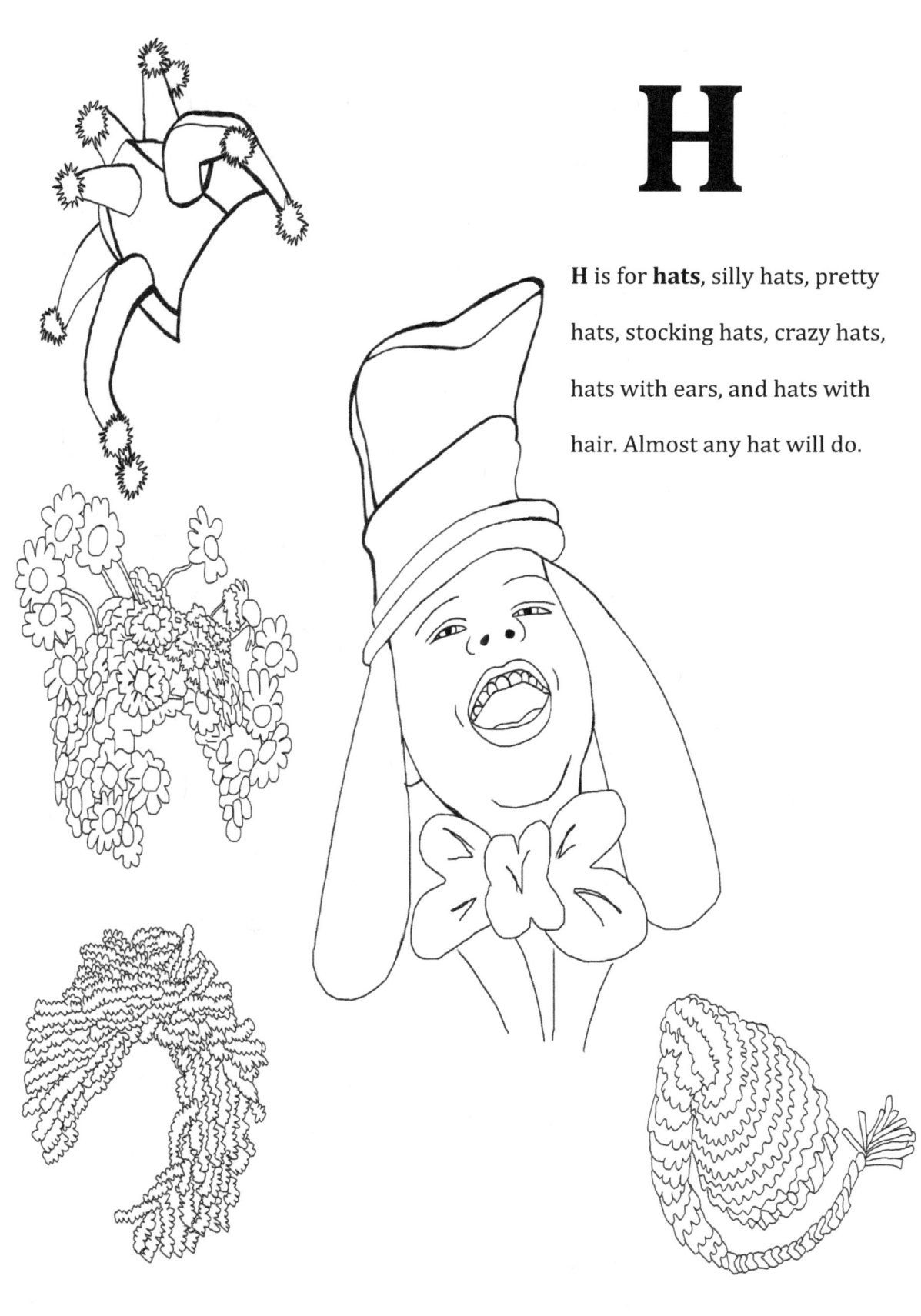

H is for **hats**, silly hats, pretty hats, stocking hats, crazy hats, hats with ears, and hats with hair. Almost any hat will do.

I is for **intravenous** lines giving me the fluids and the medicines I need to get better. The intravenous lines and the needles are my least favorite part about cancer.

I is also for **ICK**. Intravenous lines and needles can be very icky.

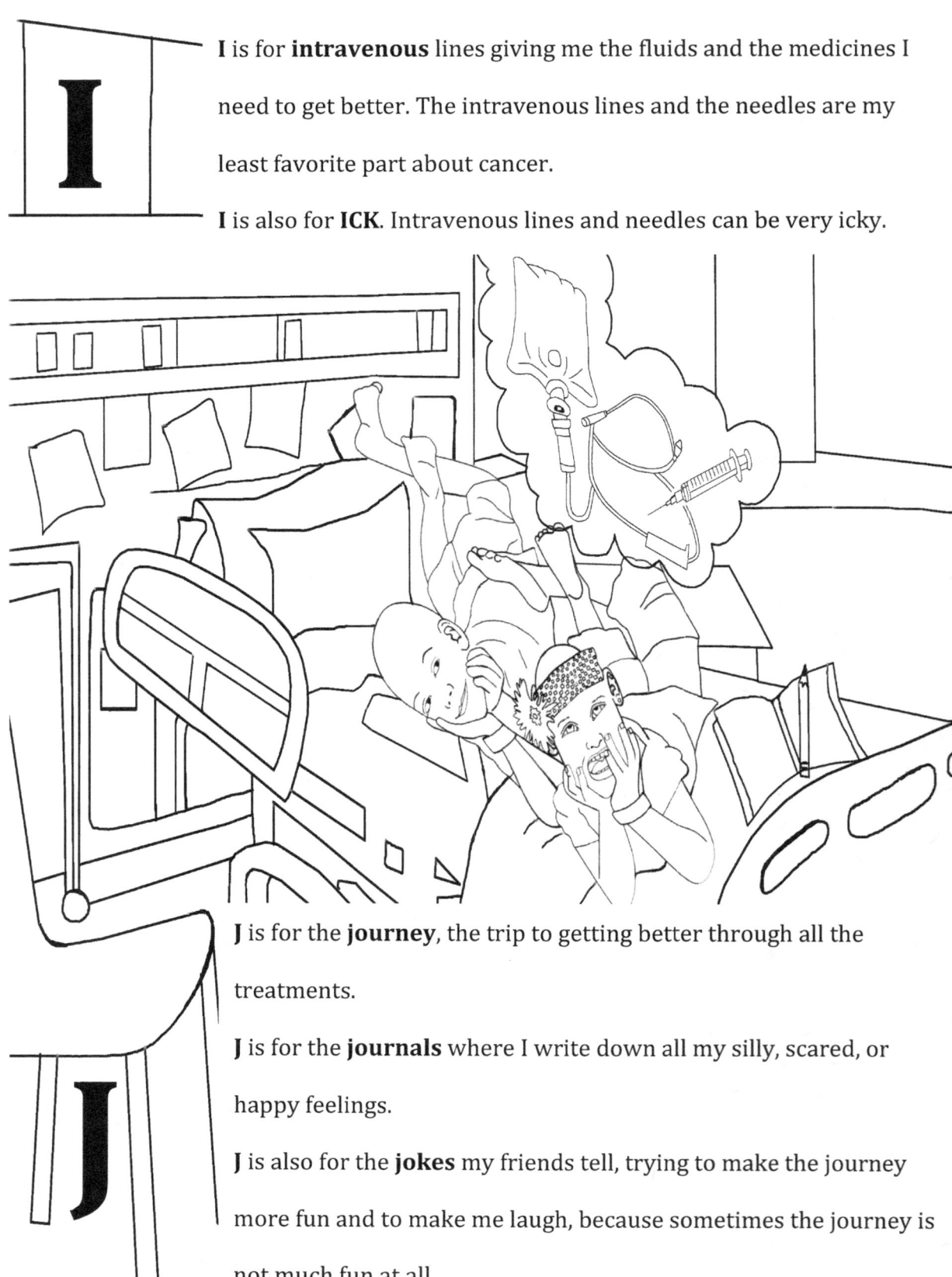

J is for the **journey**, the trip to getting better through all the treatments.

J is for the **journals** where I write down all my silly, scared, or happy feelings.

J is also for the **jokes** my friends tell, trying to make the journey more fun and to make me laugh, because sometimes the journey is not much fun at all.

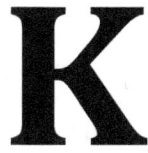

K is for **Kiwi**, my huge stuffed kangaroo that I bring to the hospital when I have to spend the night.

K is also for **knowing** that everyone loves me and is with me on my journey. I feel kind of better knowing they are on the journey, too. It still is not much fun.

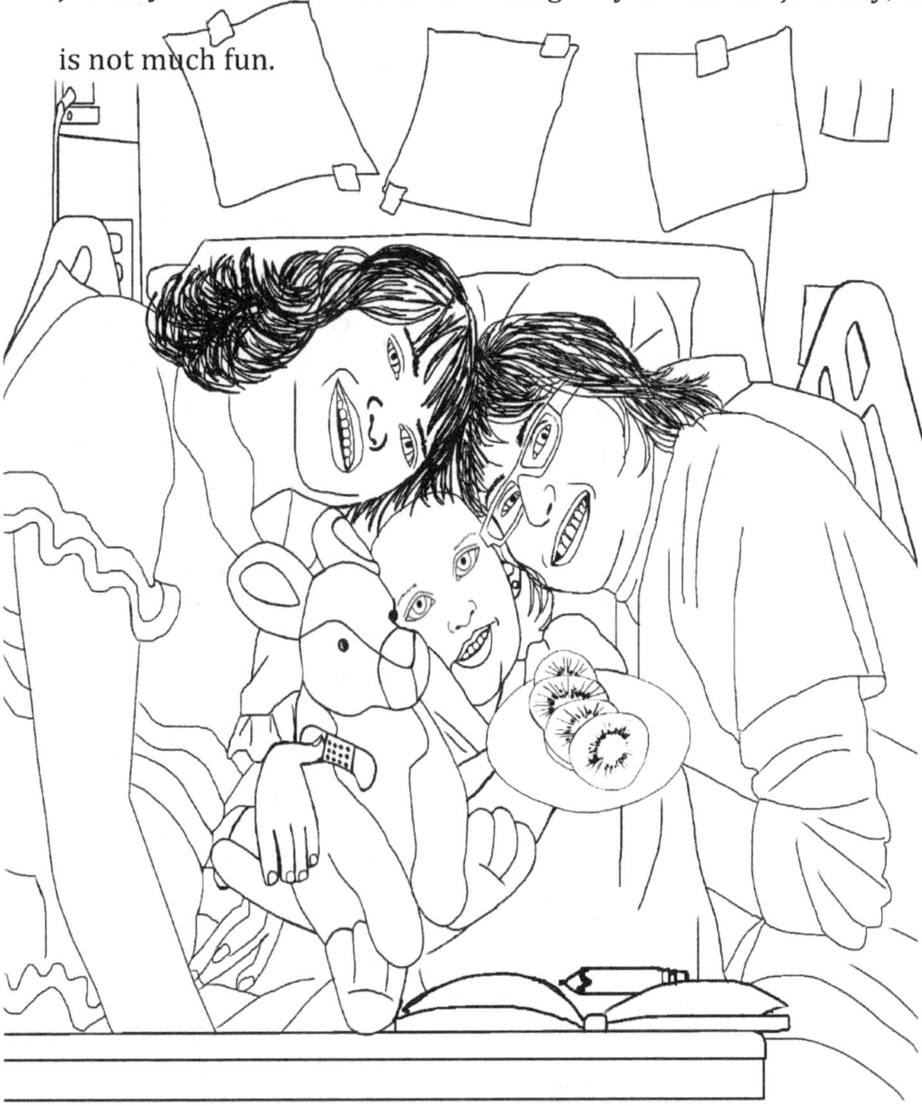

L is for **love**, lots of love from my family and friends, making me feel a lot better.

L is also for all the **letters** from kids at school who don't even know me that make me feel better, too.

M

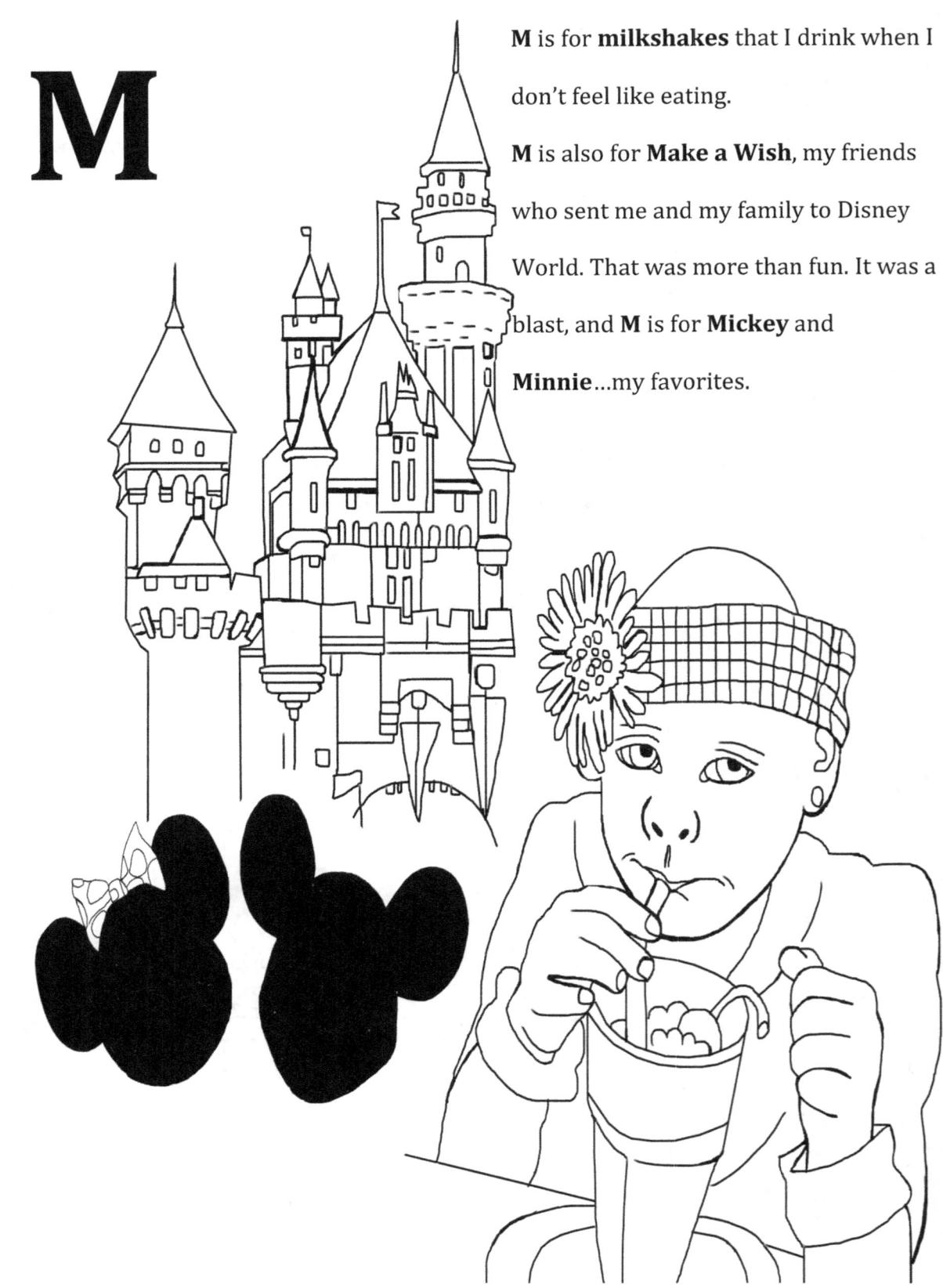

M is for **milkshakes** that I drink when I don't feel like eating.

M is also for **Make a Wish**, my friends who sent me and my family to Disney World. That was more than fun. It was a blast, and M is for **Mickey** and **Minnie**...my favorites.

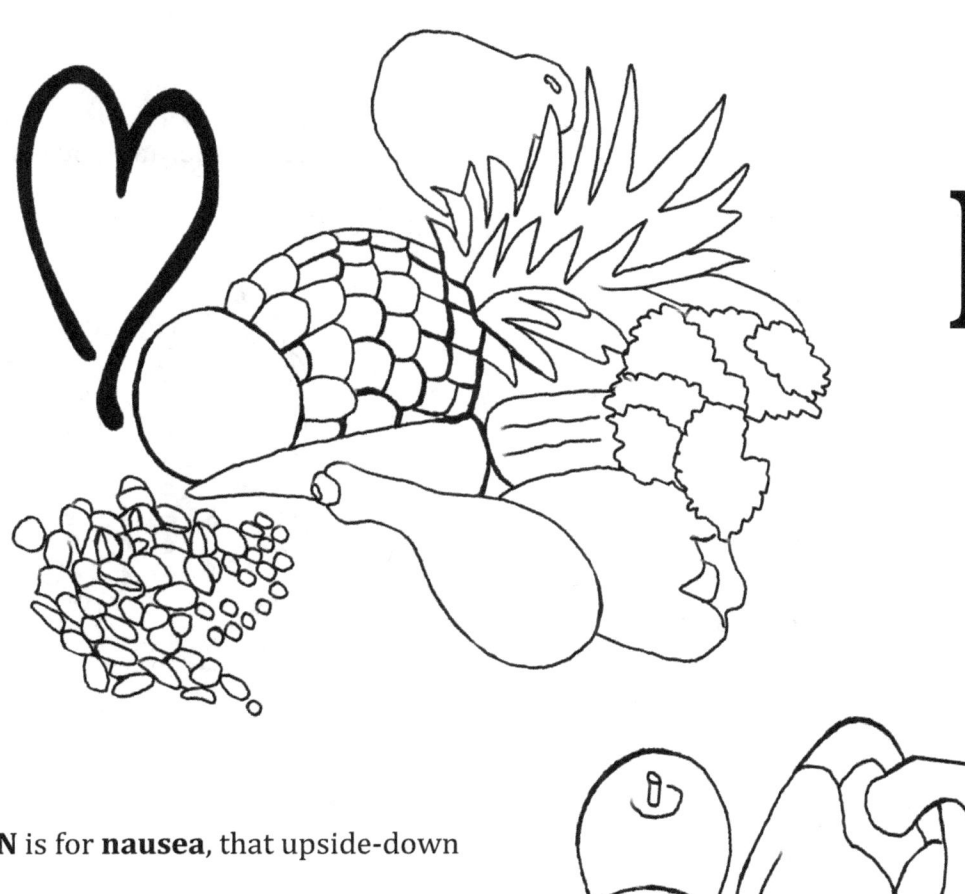

N

N is for **nausea**, that upside-down feeling flip-flopping in my tummy some days.

N is also for **nutrition**, what I need to eat to get strong, things like veggies and fruit, more milkshakes, and nuts, too.

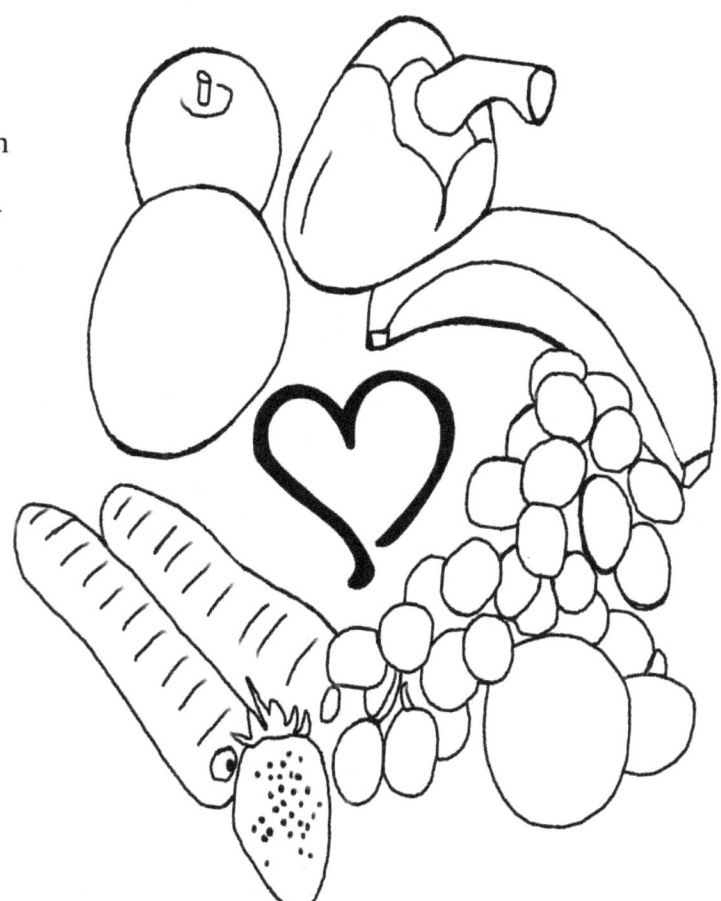

O is for **oncology**, a fancy word for the treatment of cancer.

O is also for **OUCH**, because sometimes it hurts to have cancer. I say OUCH when the nurses poke me with a needle, and once or twice I even cry. Oh well, you will have those kinds of days.

O

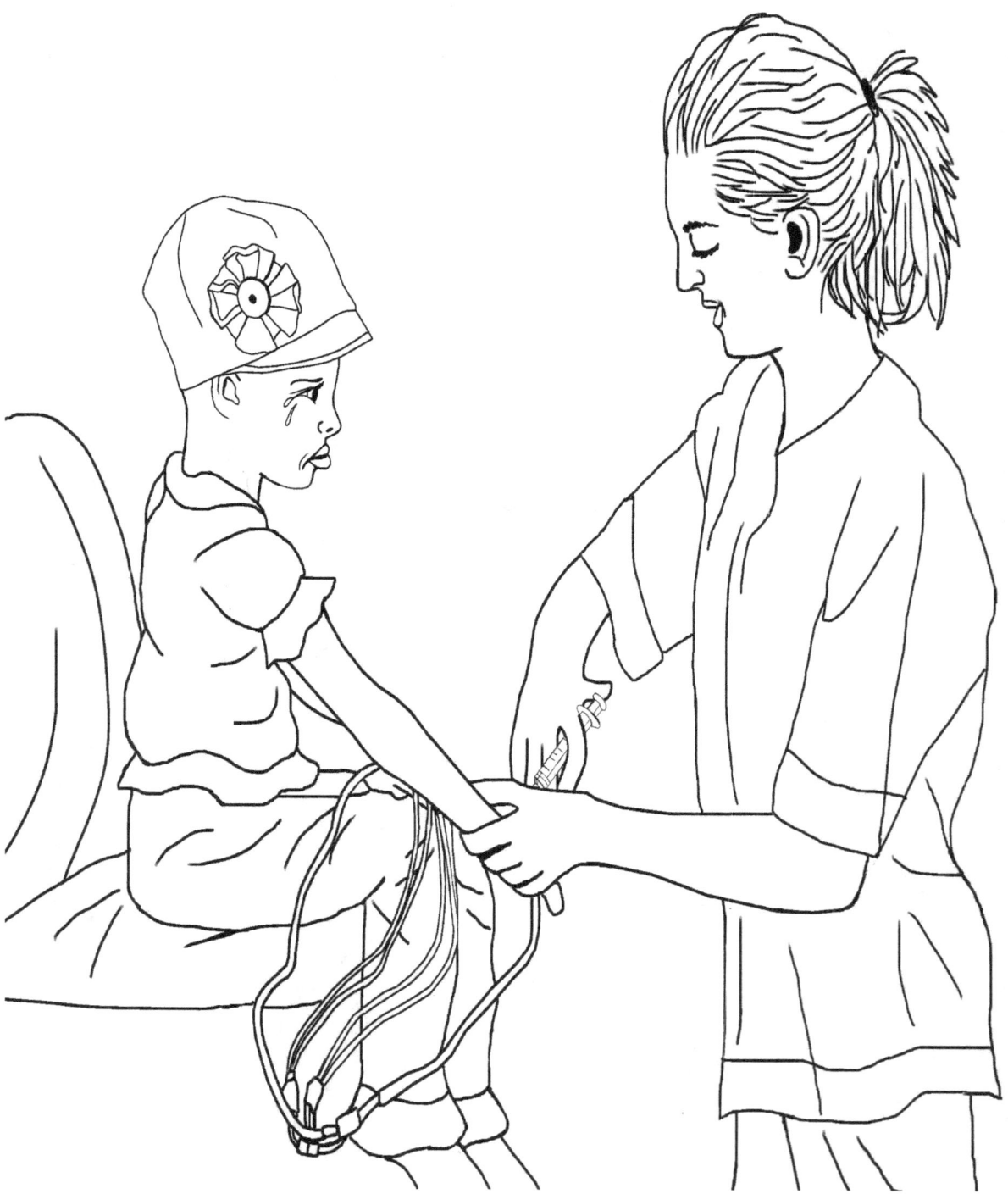

P

P is for **physician**, another fancy word for doctor. I have Dr. Amy, the best doctor ever, making me better. Everyone needs a good doctor to take care of the cancer and to be a listening friend.

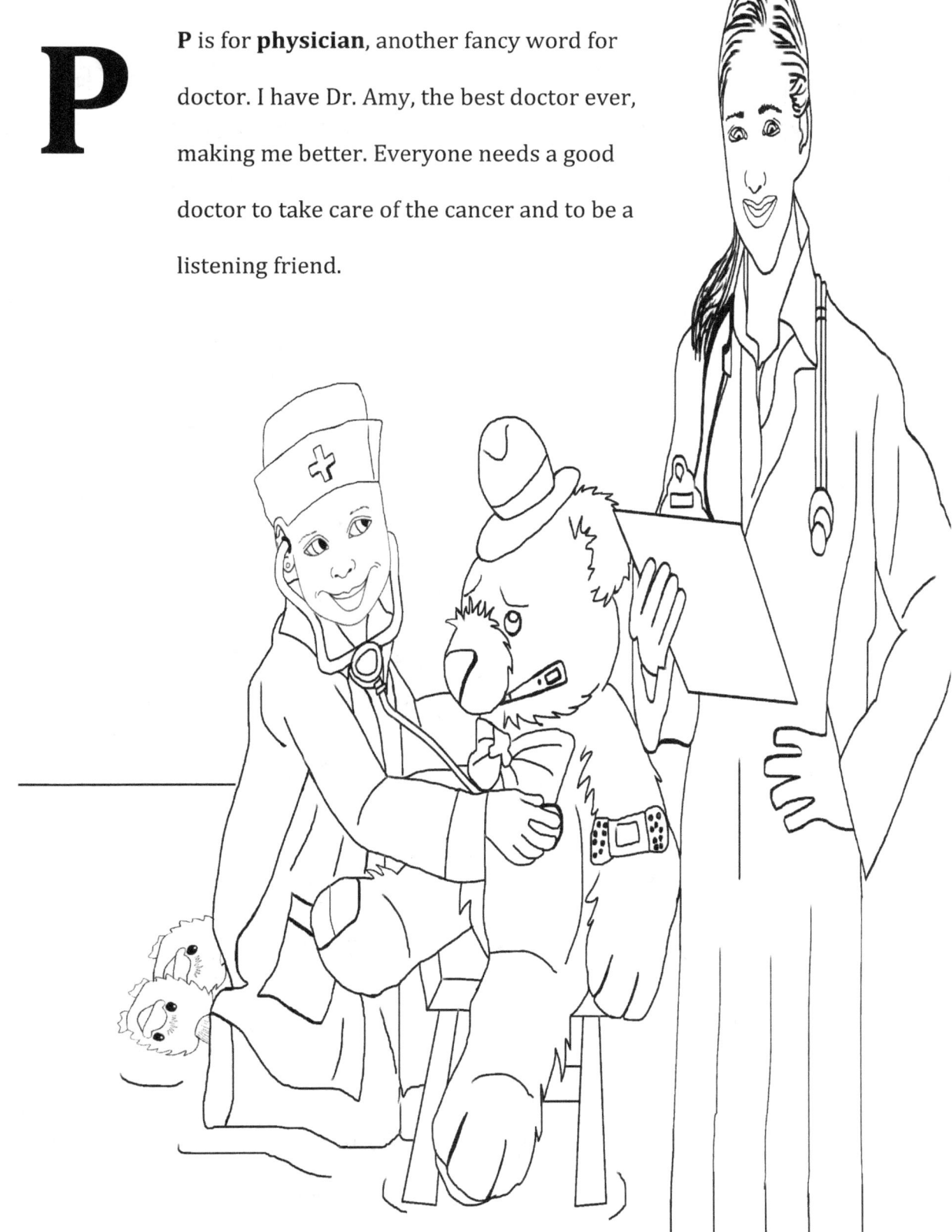

Q is for **quiet**. I put a quiet sign on my door when I want to take a nap.

Q is also for the comfy **quilt** my grandma makes to keep me warm when I nap. Someday I want to learn to sew and make kids who have cancer cozy quilts, especially those who don't have a grandma like mine.

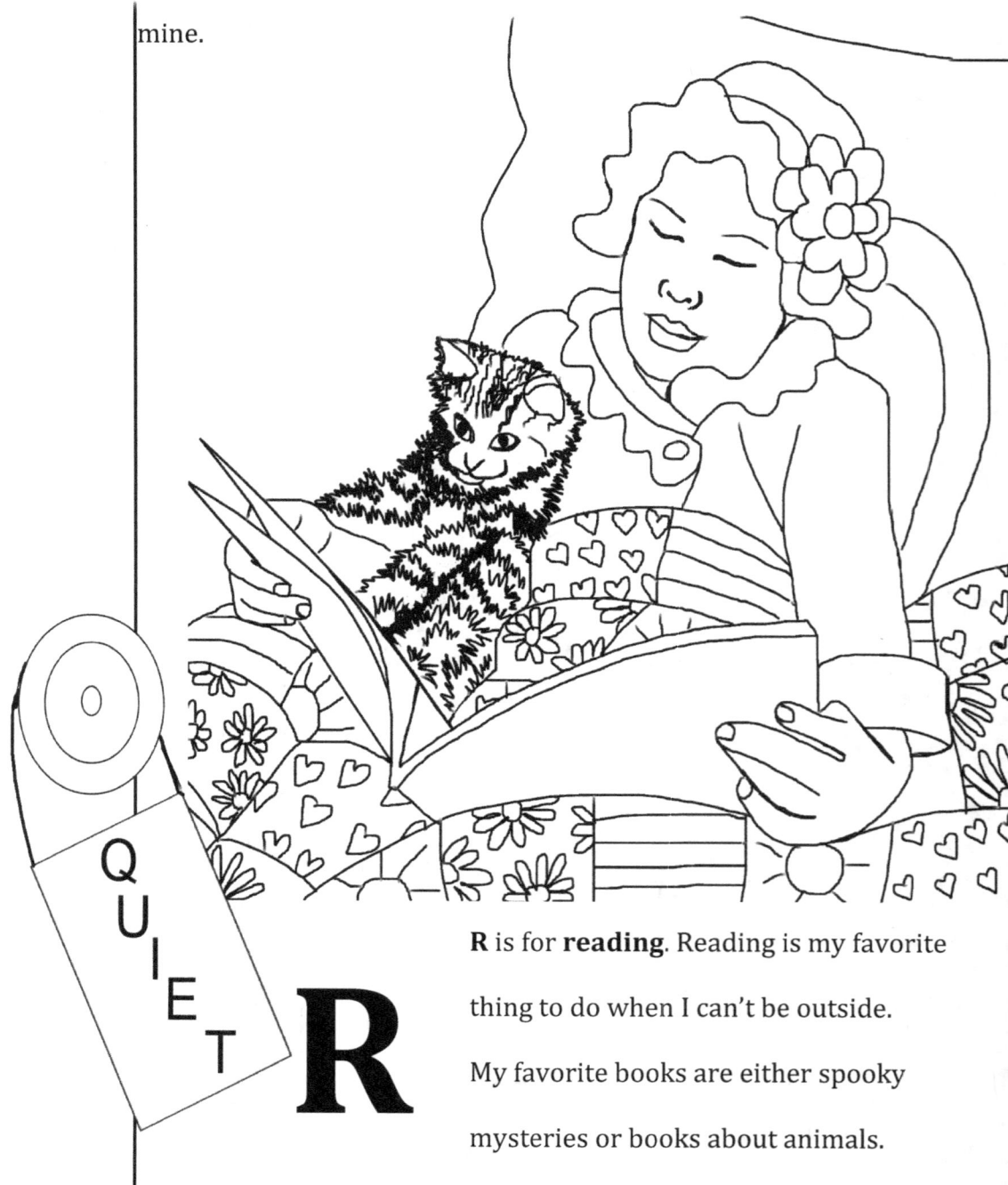

R is for **reading**. Reading is my favorite thing to do when I can't be outside. My favorite books are either spooky mysteries or books about animals.

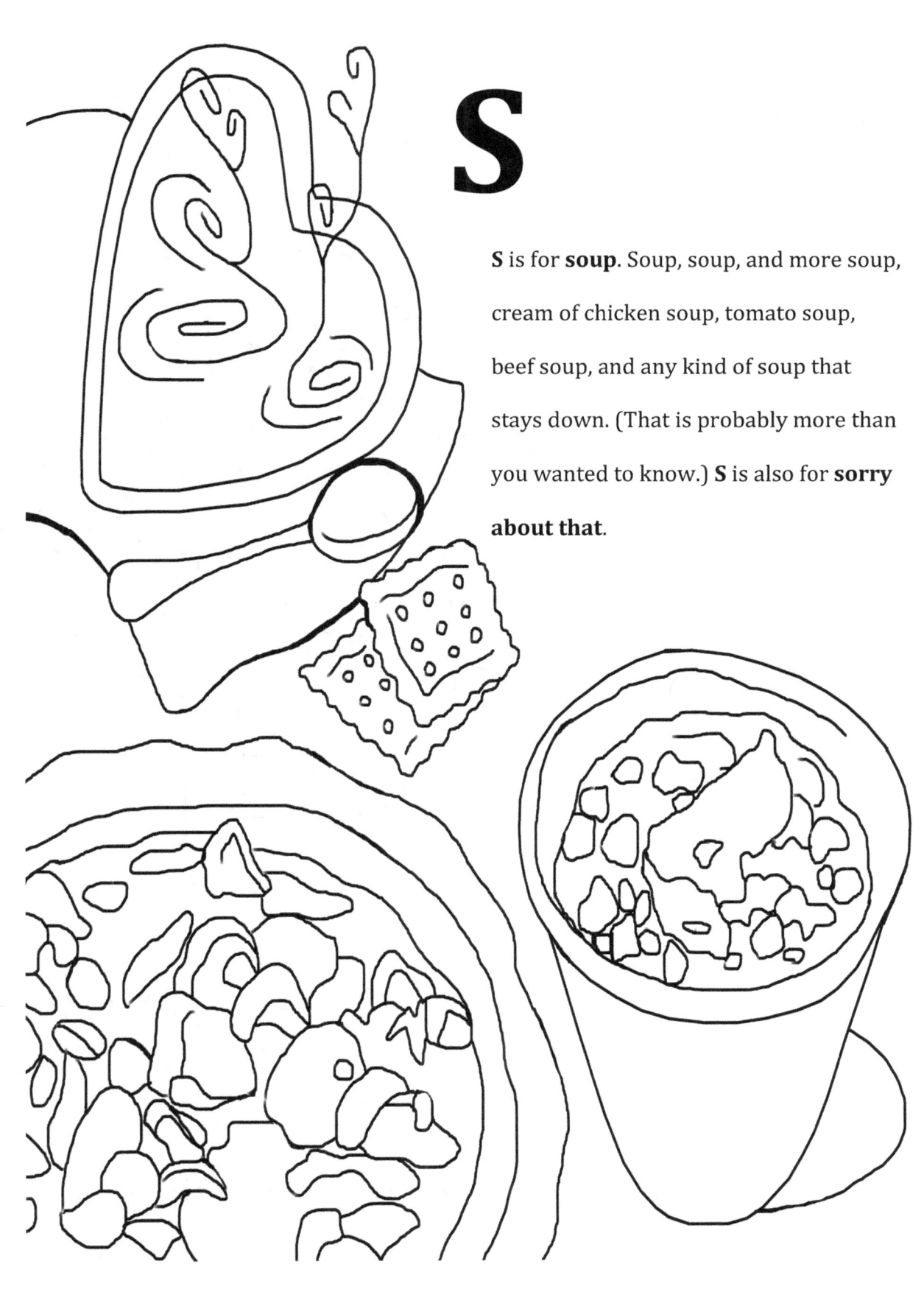

S

S is for **soup**. Soup, soup, and more soup, cream of chicken soup, tomato soup, beef soup, and any kind of soup that stays down. (That is probably more than you wanted to know.) **S** is also for **sorry about that**.

T

T is for **tests**, all of the tests I take to make sure my cancer is going away. Blood tests, ultrasound tests, urine tests, pictures of my bones kind of tests, always some kind of test—and boy do I hate

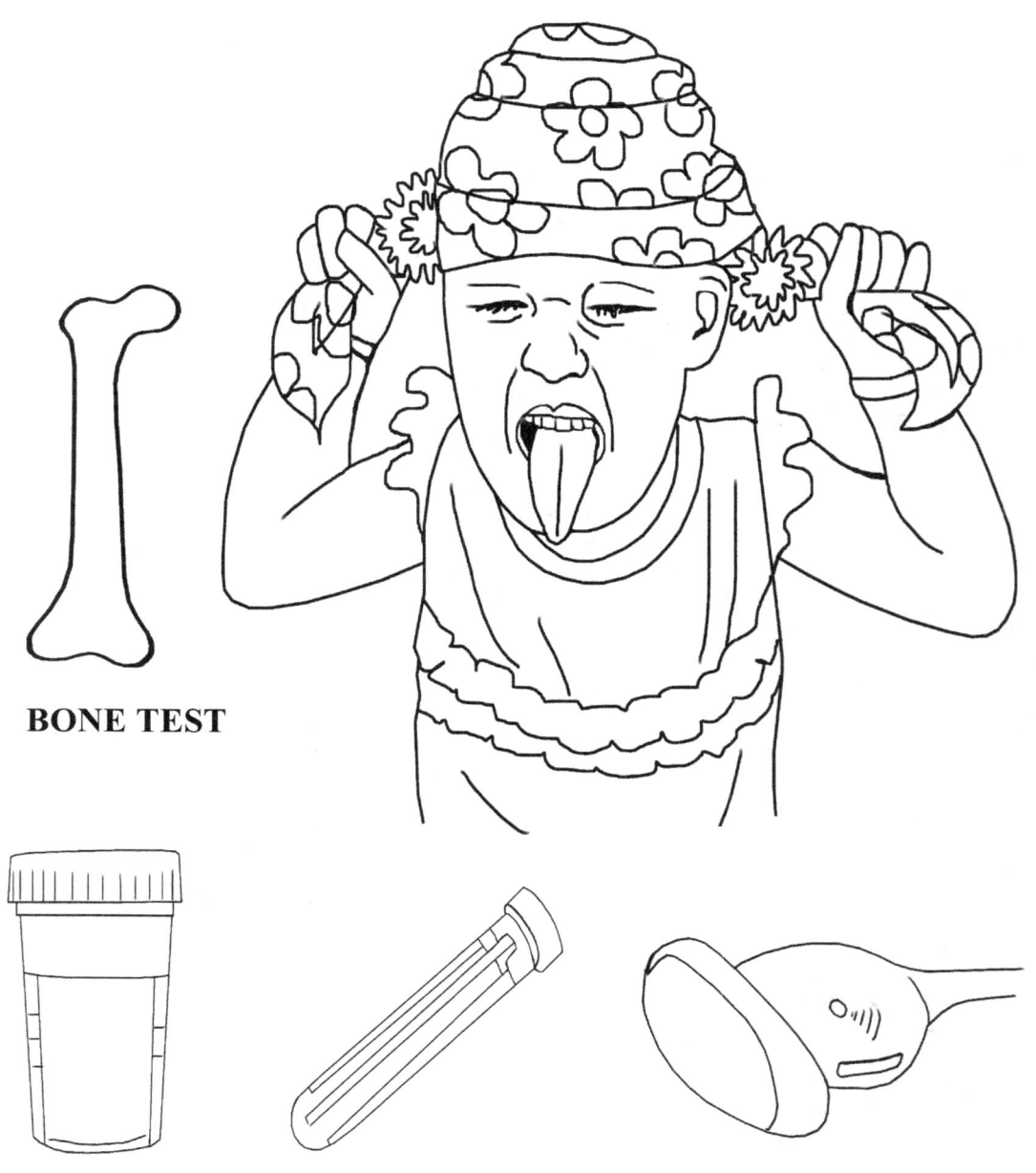

BONE TEST

URINE TEST   **BLOOD TEST**   **ULTRASOUND TEST**

U

U is for that silly **umbrella** that my mom makes me sit under to protect my skin from the sun while I am taking chemo treatments.

V

V is for the **vacation** my family and I will take to celebrate the **victory** when my leukemia is in remission. Victory is beating the enemy or success over a big obstacle. Cancer is the big obstacle, and I will win.

W

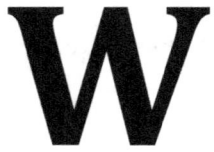

W is for the **wishes** I have.

1) to be a nurse when I grow up

2) to get a brown horse

3) to never eat Jell-O again, ever

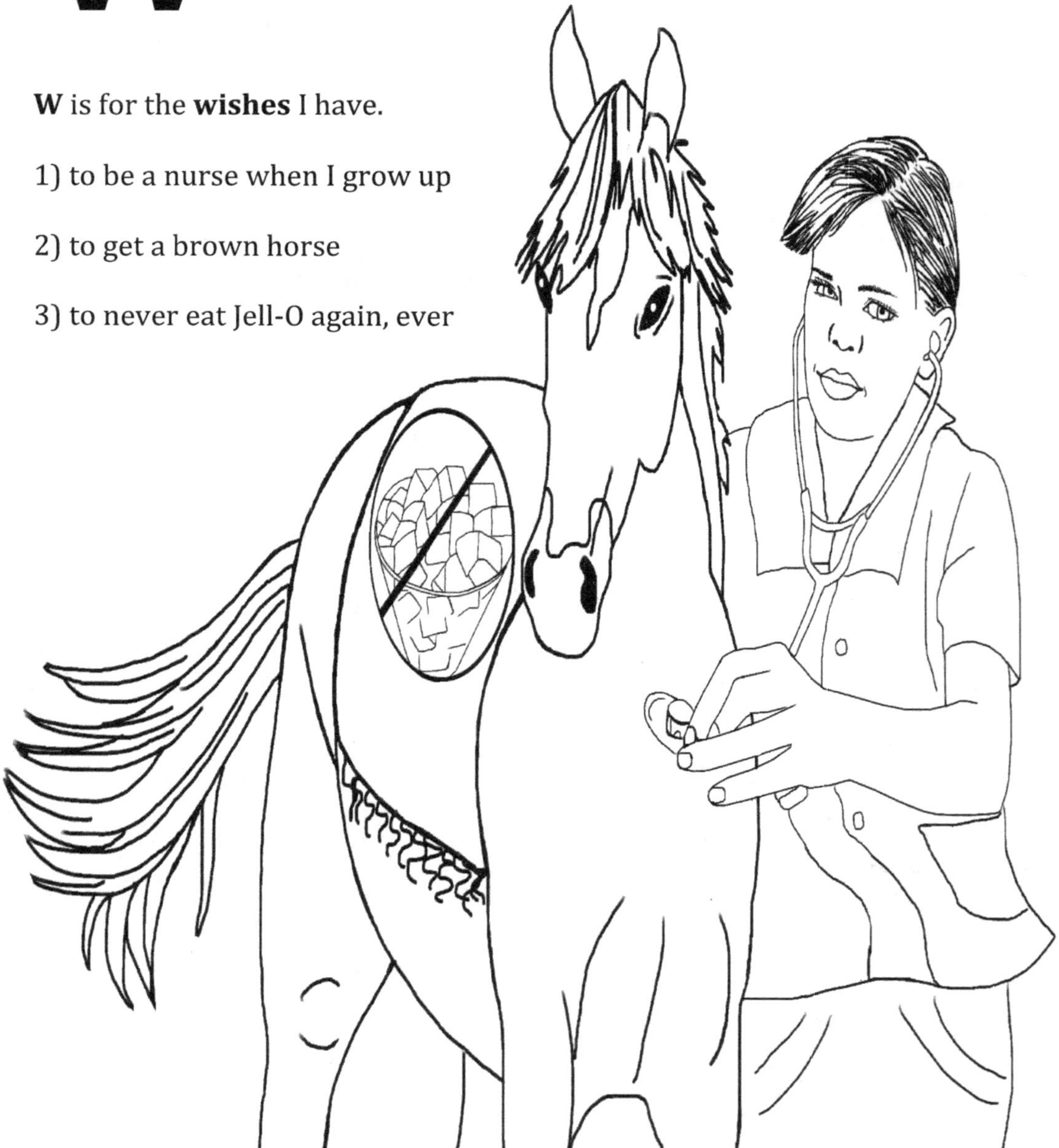

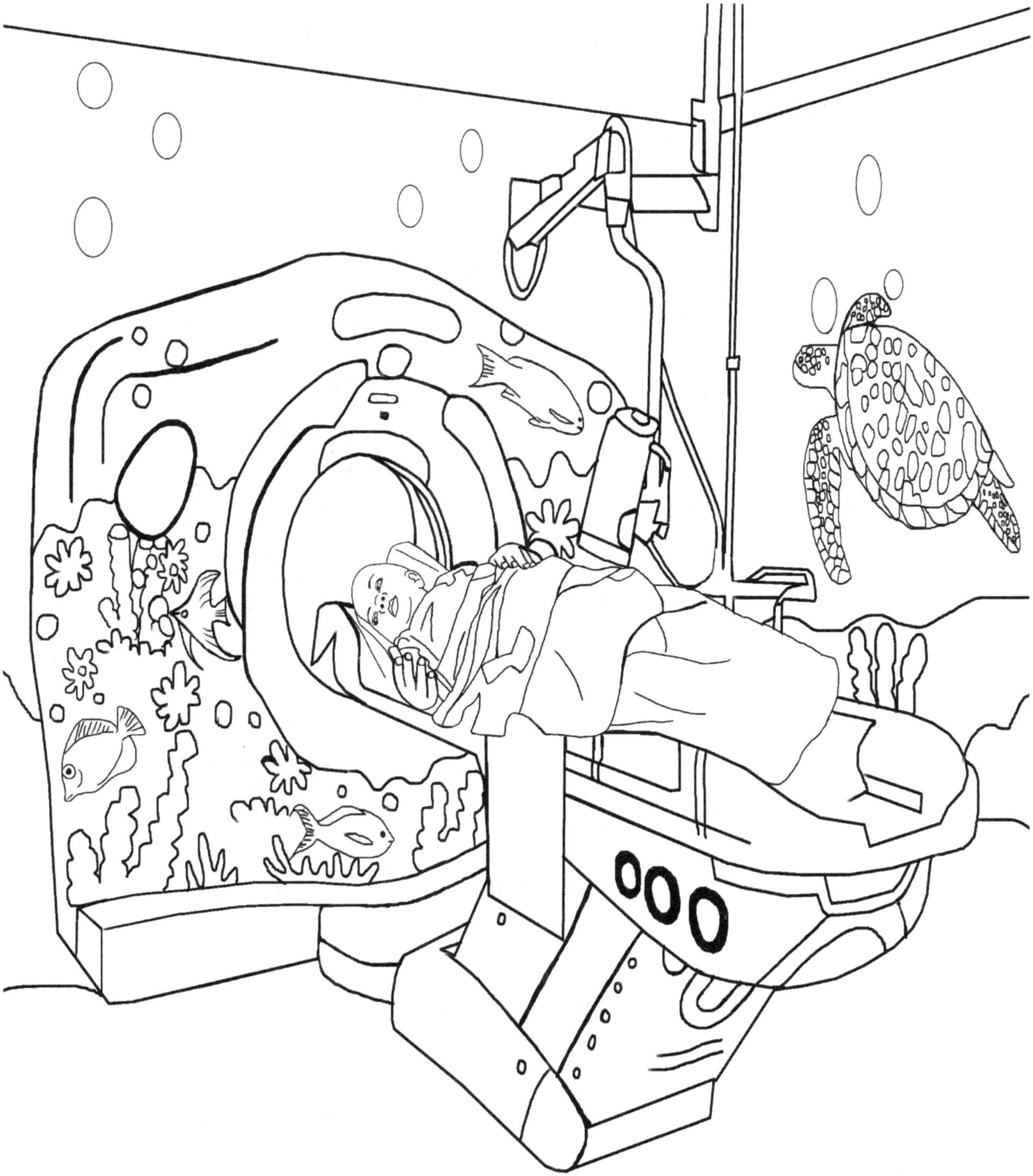

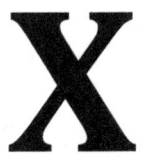

X is for **X-rays**, taking pictures of my bones and lungs to make sure the cancer is going-going-gone and not hiding somewhere we can't see.

Y

Y is for **yellow**. My favorite color reminds me of sunshine. I have yellow and pink pajamas, yellow fluffy slippers, and a yellow robe. I also have a yellow cat named Sam.

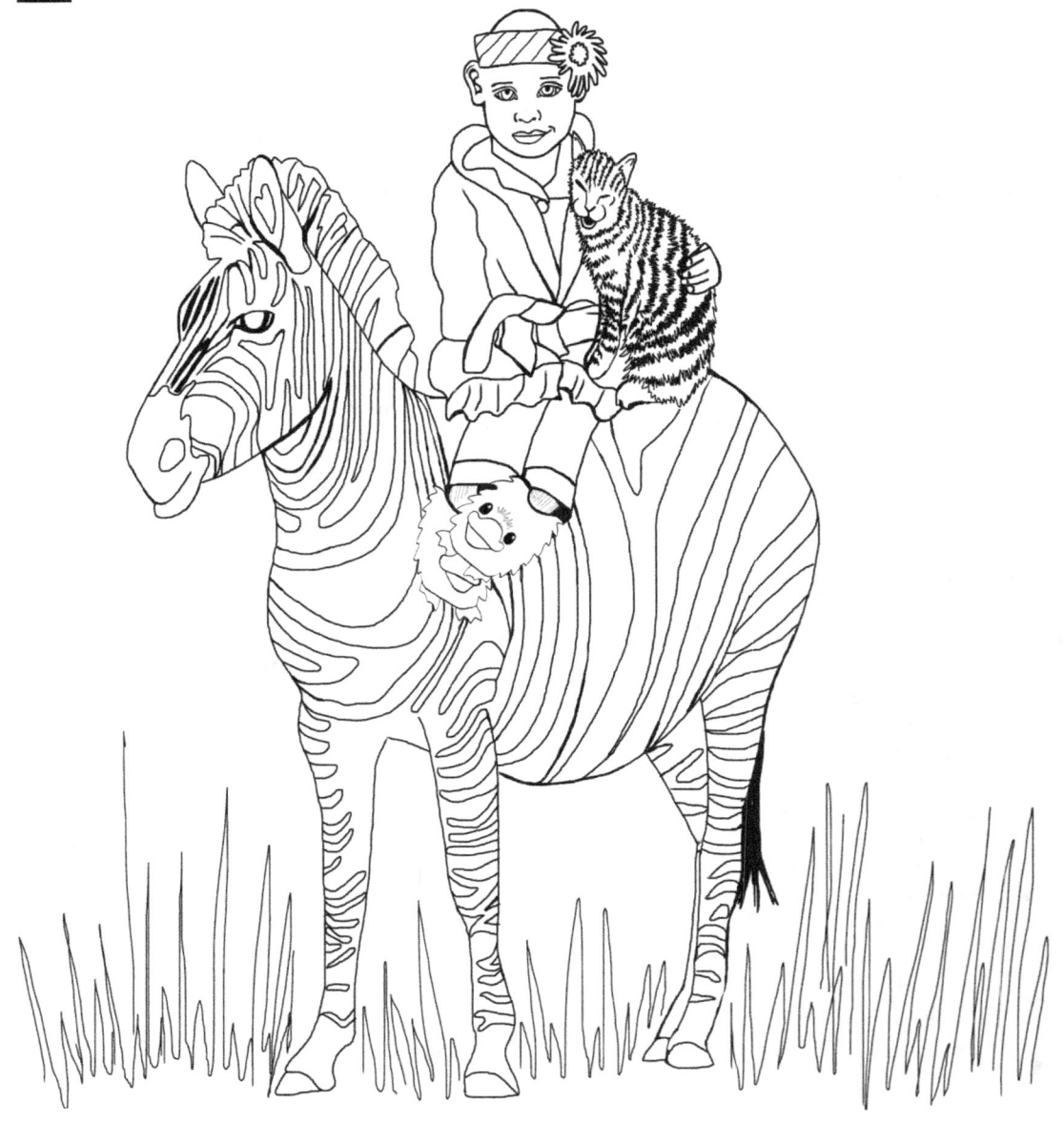

Z

Z is for **zoo**, my favorite place to visit when I feel well, and for **zebra**, the next best thing to a brown horse.

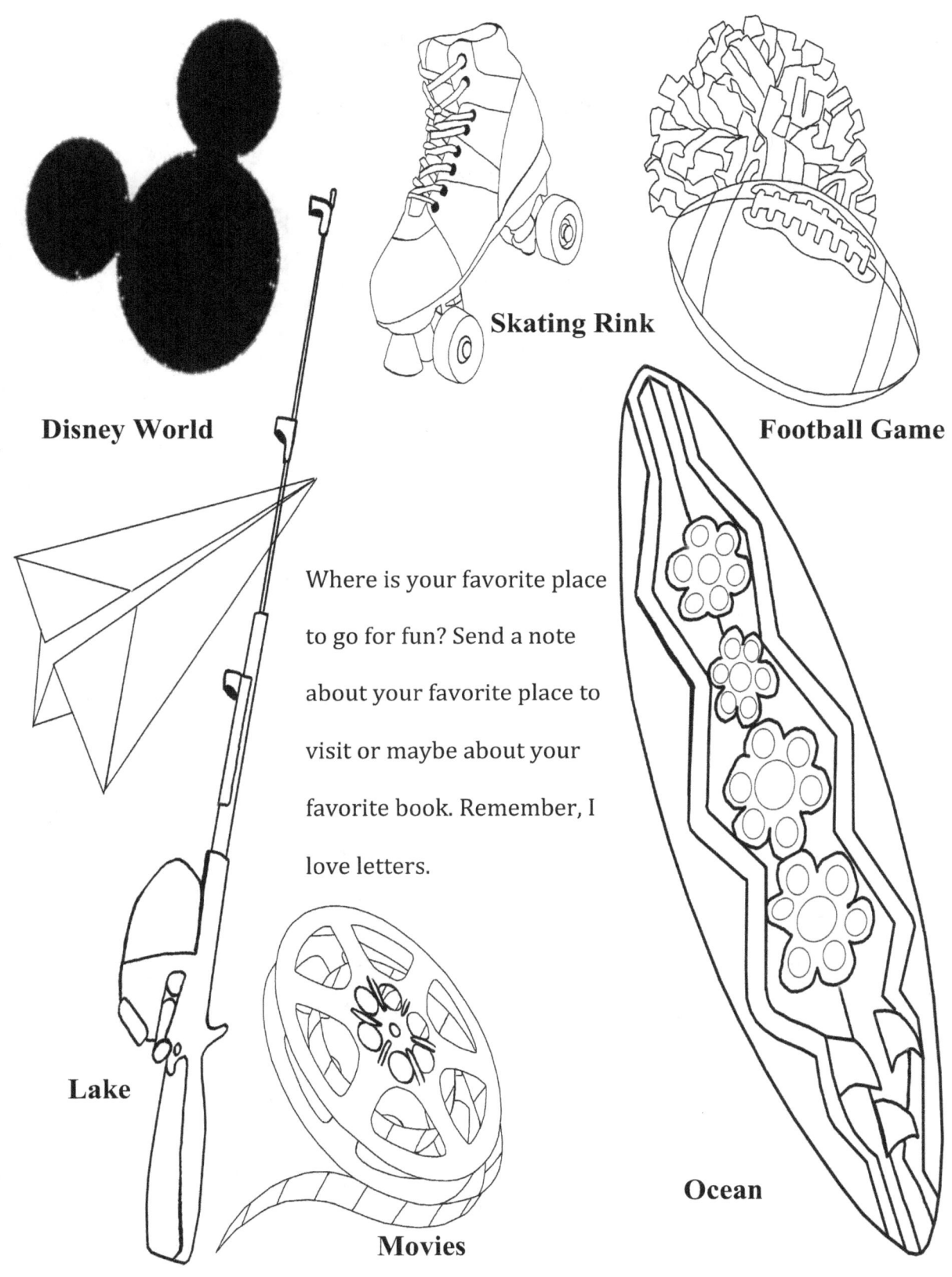

Disney World

Skating Rink

Football Game

Where is your favorite place to go for fun? Send a note about your favorite place to visit or maybe about your favorite book. Remember, I love letters.

Lake

Movies

Ocean

Ask your mom or dad to make soup for your dinner on a cold evening. Put on a crazy hat and curl up with a cup of soup and a book.

Lilly Isabella Lane's Tomato Soup

Ingredients:

1 small can crushed tomatoes, drained

1 can tomato soup

½ soup can of water

½ soup can of milk

croutons or crackers

grated cheddar cheese

salt and pepper to taste

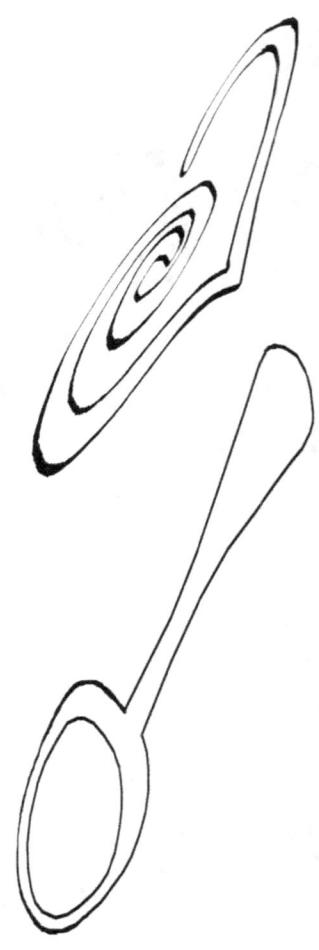

In a medium pot, mix tomatoes with tomato soup, water and milk until smooth. Heat the mixture on top of the stove until desired temperature. My mom makes a double batch and heats it in the crock pot for a couple hours. Then it is ready when anyone wants a cup.

Serve in a cup or bowl. Top with croutons or crackers and grated cheese. It is oh so good.

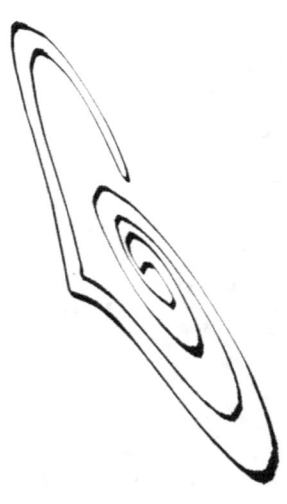

Lilly Isabella Lane's Cream of Chicken Soup

Ingredients:

2 C cooked white chicken, chopped

4 packets Lipton's Cream of Chicken Cup of Soup or four

chicken bouillon seasoning packets

1 can of chicken broth

2 tsp flour

2 tsp margarine

3-4 C milk

1 stalk celery, chopped

sprinkle of onion powder

salt and pepper to taste

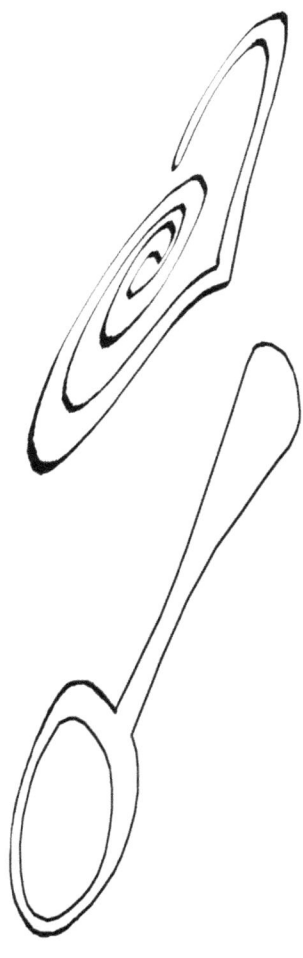

Combine margarine, celery and flour in a saucepan and melt over medium heat. Slowly stir in the broth. Mix in the four soup packets and stir. Slowly add milk to make the soup the consistency you desire. Add chicken. Simmer on low heat until thickened and smooth. My mom adds a little more flour or another packet of soup mix if it looks too runny. Add salt and pepper to taste. Enjoy. It's pretty yummy.

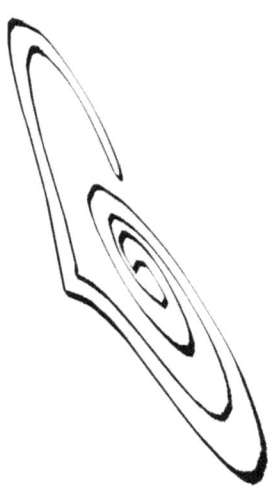

www.ingramcontent.com/pod-product-compliance
Lightning Source LLC
Chambersburg PA
CBHW081152290526
45795CB00008B/2893